DIETARY SOLUTION FOR BLOOD SUGAR CONTROL

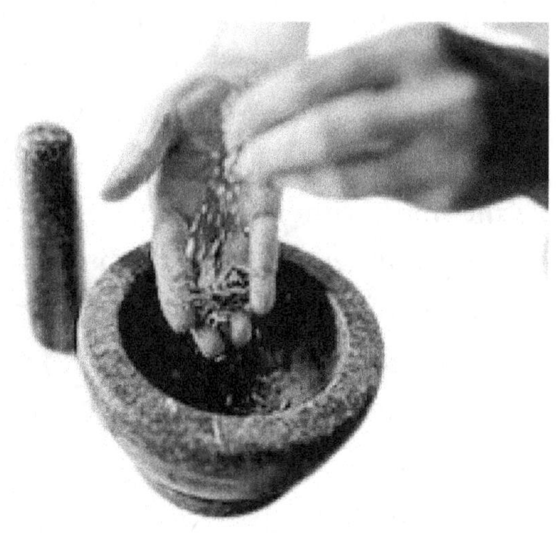

The ultimate guide to controlling blood sugar through diet

Deon flames

Copyright © 2023 by Deon flames

Table of Contents

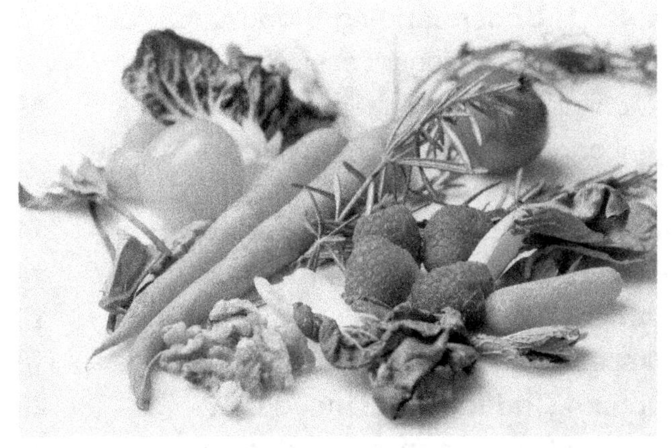

Introduction

Once upon a time, in a small town nestled between rolling hills, lived a woman named Emily. Struggling with erratic blood sugar levels for years, she stumbled upon an old, dusty book in the town's quaint library. The title, "Harmony Within: A Guide to Balancing Your Body."
Intrigued, Emily delved into the pages, discovering a wealth of knowledge about holistic approaches to health. The author emphasized the power of mindful eating, regular exercise, and the influence of stress on the body. Emily embraced these teachings, transforming her lifestyle.
With dedication, she incorporated wholesome foods and adopted a daily exercise routine. The book's guidance on stress management proved invaluable, leading Emily to explore meditation and relaxation techniques. As weeks passed, her blood sugar levels stabilized, and she felt a renewed sense of vitality. Word of Emily's success spread throughout the town, inspiring others to explore alternative paths to health. The once-forgotten book became a beacon of hope, as more individuals sought its wisdom. In time, the community transformed into a haven for holistic well-being, all thanks to a chance discovery and one woman's determination to rewrite her health story. Welcome to "Balancing Act: A Comprehensive Guide to Managing Blood Sugar Levels Through Diet." In the ever-evolving landscape of health and wellness, understanding

the intricate relationship between dietary choices and blood sugar regulation is paramount. This book serves as your compass on a journey towards stable blood sugar levels, offering not just a collection of recipes, but a holistic approach that combines nutritional insights, lifestyle adjustments, and practical strategies.

In the pages ahead, we delve into the science behind blood sugar, unraveling the mysteries of glycemic index, insulin response, and how various foods impact glucose levels. From there, we transition into a practical guide, providing you with a roadmap for crafting a personalized and sustainable dietary plan. Discover the power of nutrient-dense whole foods, explore mindful eating practices, and learn how to make informed choices that foster a healthy glycemic profile.

Our aim is not only to empower you with knowledge but to inspire lasting change. We understand the challenges of maintaining balanced blood sugar in today's fast-paced world, and our approach is rooted in practicality. Whether you're seeking to prevent diabetes, manage existing conditions, or simply optimize your well-being, "Balancing Act" is your companion for navigating the intricate interplay between nutrition and blood sugar control.

Embark on this transformative journey with us, and unlock the potential of a diet that not only nourishes your body but also harmonizes your blood sugar levels. Your path to vibrant health starts here.

Chapter 1: Understanding Blood Sugar Levels

Blood sugar levels, also known as blood glucose levels, play a crucial role in maintaining overall health. Glucose, derived from the food we consume, serves as the primary source of energy for our cells. Understanding blood sugar levels is essential for managing various health conditions, particularly diabetes.

Normal Blood Sugar Levels:

Fasting Blood Sugar: Typically measured after atleast 8 hours of fasting, normal levels are around 70-100 mg/dL.

Postprandial Blood Sugar: Measured 1-2 hours after a meal, normal levels are below 140 mg/dL.

Regulation of Blood Sugar:

Insulin: Produced by the pancreas, insulin helps cells absorb glucose from the bloodstream, reducing blood sugar levels.

Glucagon: Released by the pancreas, it raises blood sugar levels by prompting the liver to convert stored glycogen into glucose.

Factors Influencing Blood Sugar Levels:

Diet: Carbohydrates have the most significant impact on blood sugar. Managing carbohydrate intake is crucial.

Physical Activity: Exercise enhances insulin sensitivity, helping regulate blood sugar levels.

Stress: Stress hormones can elevate blood sugar levels. Chronic stress may contribute to long-term imbalances.

Type 1 Diabetes: Resulting from the immune system attacking insulin-producing cells, individuals with Type 1 diabetes require insulin injections.

Type 2 Diabetes: Often linked to lifestyle factors, the body becomes resistant to insulin. Management involves lifestyle changes, medication, or insulin.

Monitoring Blood Sugar Levels:

Blood Glucose Meters: Portable devices used by individuals with diabetes to monitor their blood sugar levels.

Continuous Glucose Monitoring (CGM): Provides real-time data on blood sugar levels, offering better insights for diabetes management.

Complications of High Blood Sugar:

Hyperglycemia: Prolonged high blood sugar levels can lead to symptoms such as increased thirst, frequent urination, and fatigue.

Complications: Uncontrolled diabetes can result in serious complications, including cardiovascular issues, kidney problems, and nerve damage.

Preventing and Managing Imbalances:

Healthy Diet: Focus on a balanced diet with an emphasis on whole grains, fruits, vegetables, lean proteins, and healthy fats.

Regular Exercise: Physical activity aids in weight management and improves insulin sensitivity.

Medication: For individuals with diabetes, medications or insulin may be prescribed to regulate blood sugar.

Regular Check-ups:Routine monitoring and regular check-ups with healthcare professionals are essential for individuals with diabetes to adjust treatment plans as needed.

Understanding blood sugar levels involves a holistic approach to lifestyle, diet, and medical management. It is crucial for both preventing the onset of diabetes and effectively managing the condition for those already diagnosed.

Importance of Maintaining Balanced Blood Sugar

Maintaining balanced blood sugar levels is crucial for overall health and well-being. The body relies on a stable glucose concentration in the bloodstream to fuel its cells and organs. Here are several key reasons why it is important to keep blood sugar levels in check:

Energy Regulation: Balanced blood sugar levels ensure a steady and consistent supply of energy to the body's cells, tissues, and organs. This helps prevent energy crashes and fatigue, promoting sustained physical and mental performance throughout the day.

Weight Management: Fluctuations in blood sugar can contribute to overeating and weight gain. When blood sugar levels spike, the body may release excess insulin, leading to increased fat storage. Conversely, low blood sugar levels can trigger cravings for quick energy sources, often resulting in the consumption of unhealthy snacks.

Diabetes Prevention: Persistent high blood sugar levels are a hallmark of diabetes. By maintaining balanced blood sugar, individuals can reduce their risk of developing type 2 diabetes. Regular monitoring and healthy lifestyle choices, such as a balanced diet and regular exercise, play crucial roles in diabetes prevention.

Heart Health: Elevated blood sugar levels can contribute to cardiovascular problems. It is associated with an increased risk of heart disease, including conditions like atherosclerosis and coronary artery disease. Managing blood sugar levels can contribute to overall heart health.

Mood and Mental Health: Blood sugar imbalances can impact mood and cognitive function. Rapid drops or spikes in glucose levels may lead to irritability, difficulty concentrating, and mood swings. Sustaining stable blood sugar levels supports better emotional well-being and mental clarity.

Preventing Hypoglycemia: On the flip side, low blood sugar (hypoglycemia) can be equally problematic. It can cause symptoms such as dizziness, confusion, and, in severe cases, unconsciousness. Maintaining a balanced blood sugar level helps prevent hypoglycemic episodes.

Improved Insulin Sensitivity: Balanced blood sugar levels contribute to better insulin sensitivity. This means that the body's cells respond effectively to insulin, the hormone responsible for regulating blood sugar. Improved insulin sensitivity lowers the risk of insulin resistance and type 2 diabetes.

Long-term Health: Chronic imbalances in blood sugar can contribute to various health issues, including nerve damage, kidney problems, and vision impairment. By managing blood sugar levels, individuals can mitigate the risk of developing these serious complications.

maintaining balanced blood sugar is a fundamental aspect of a healthy lifestyle. It not only helps prevent immediate issues like fatigue and mood swings but also plays a crucial role in preventing long-term health complications. Adopting a well-rounded approach, including a balanced diet, regular physical activity, and stress management, is key to promoting stable blood sugar levels and overall well-being.

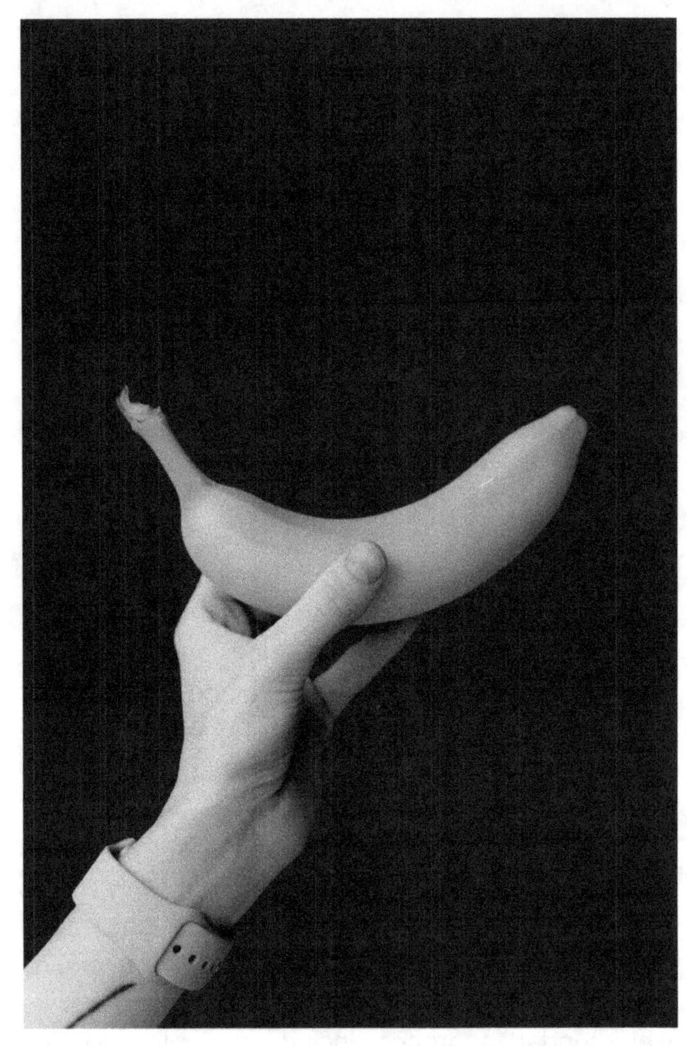

Chapter 2 Fundamentals of Nutrition –

Macronutrients and Micronutrients

Nutrition is the science that explores how the body uses the nutrients found in food for growth, maintenance, and overall well-being. The fundamental components of nutrition include macronutrients and micronutrients.

1. **Macronutrients**:
    - Carbohydrates: These are the body's primary source of energy. They can be simple (sugars) or complex (starches and fibers). Good sources include fruits, vegetables, whole grains, and legumes.
    - Proteins: Essential for the repair and maintenance of tissues, proteins are composed of amino

acids. Sources of protein include meat, dairy products, eggs, legumes, and nuts.

- Fats: Fats are crucial for energy storage, cell structure, and the absorption of fat-soluble vitamins (A, D, E, and K). Healthy fat sources include avocados, nuts, seeds, olive oil, and fatty fish.

2. **Micronutrients**:

- Vitamins: Essential for various biochemical processes, vitamins are classified as water-soluble (e.g., B-vitamins, vitamin C) or fat-soluble (e.g., vitamin A, D, E, K). They are found in a variety of foods, including fruits, vegetables, dairy, and meat.
- Minerals: These inorganic nutrients are critical for various physiological functions. Examples include calcium for bone health, iron for oxygen transport, and potassium for fluid balance. Sources of minerals vary and include dairy, leafy greens, meats, and nuts.

3. **Water**:

- o Often overlooked, water is a fundamental nutrient vital for hydration and the proper functioning of bodily processes. It plays a role in digestion, nutrient transport, and temperature regulation. Adequate water intake is essential for overall health.

4. **Dietary Guidelines**:
    - o Dietary recommendations vary based on factors such as age, sex, activity level, and health status. A balanced diet, comprising a variety of foods from different food groups, is generally advised.

5. **Nutritional Requirements**:
    - o Individual nutritional needs depend on factors like age, sex, weight, height, and physical activity. Adequate intake of nutrients is crucial for preventing deficiencies and promoting optimal health.

6. **Nutritional Disorders**:
    - o Malnutrition can result from an imbalance of nutrients, leading to deficiencies or excesses. Conditions like obesity, diabetes,

and cardiovascular diseases are often linked to poor dietary habits.

7. **Nutrition and Health**:
    - A well-balanced diet is fundamental for maintaining overall health and preventing chronic diseases. It contributes to proper growth and development, immune function, and cognitive performance.

Understanding the fundamentals of nutrition empowers individuals to make informed dietary choices, promoting a healthy and fulfilling lifestyle. Always consult with healthcare professionals or registered dietitians for personalized nutritional advice.

Chapter 3 Glycemic Index Demystified

The Glycemic Index (GI) measures how quickly a carbohydrate-containing food raises blood glucose levels. Foods with a high GI are rapidly digested and cause a quicker spike in blood sugar, while low-GI foods are absorbed more slowly, leading to a gradual and steady blood sugar increase.

Impact of Different Foods on Blood Sugar

Certainly! Different foods affect blood sugar levels differently. Here's a brief overview:

Carbohydrates: Foods rich in carbohydrates, such as bread, rice, and pasta, can cause a rapid increase in blood sugar levels. Simple carbohydrates like sugary snacks can lead to a quicker spike than complex carbohydrates found in whole grains.

Proteins: Protein-rich foods have a minimal impact on blood sugar levels. They are slower to digest and absorb, providing a more gradual and sustained release of glucose.

Fats: Fats also have a minimal immediate impact on blood sugar. However, a high-fat meal can delay the absorption of carbohydrates, affecting blood sugar levels over a more extended period.

Fiber: Foods high in fiber, like fruits, vegetables, and whole grains, can help stabilize blood sugar levels. Fiber slows down the digestion and absorption of carbohydrates, preventing rapid spikes.

Glycemic Index (GI): The glycemic index measures how quickly a particular food raises blood sugar. Foods with a high GI cause a rapid increase, while those with a low GI result in a slower, more gradual rise.

Balancing the types and amounts of carbohydrates, including fiber-rich foods, along with proteins and healthy fats, can contribute to better blood sugar management, especially for individuals with diabetes or those looking to maintain stable energy levels.

Chapter 4 Crafting a Balanced Diet

Crafting a balanced diet is crucial in managing diabetes and promoting overall health. By incorporating a mix of complex carbohydrates, lean proteins, healthy fats, and fiber, you can help regulate blood sugar levels and support sustained energy throughout the day. It's essential to pay attention to portion sizes, choose nutrient-dense foods, and spread meals and snacks evenly to maintain stability in blood glucose levels and as such we'll be delving into crafting balanced diet for blood sugar control below:

Complex Carbohydrates: Choose whole grains, legumes, and vegetables for a slow release of sugar into the bloodstream, helping to maintain stable blood sugar levels.

Protein Sources: Include lean proteins like poultry, fish, tofu, and legumes to promote satiety and support muscle health.

Healthy Fats: Opt for sources of unsaturated fats, such as avocados, nuts, and olive oil, which can help regulate blood sugar and provide long-lasting energy.

Fiber-Rich Foods: Increase fiber intake with fruits, vegetables, and whole grains to slow digestion and improve blood sugar control.

Portion Control: Manage portion sizes to avoid overeating, helping to prevent rapid spikes in blood sugar levels.

Regular Meals: Establish a consistent eating schedule with balanced meals and snacks to regulate blood sugar throughout the day.

Limit Added Sugars: Minimize consumption of sugary beverages, sweets, and processed foods to prevent sudden blood sugar spikes.

Hydration: Stay well-hydrated with water, as dehydration can affect blood sugar levels. Limit sugary drinks and alcohol.

Balanced Snacks: Choose snacks with a combination of protein and fiber to maintain energy levels between meals.

Monitor Carbohydrate Intake: Be mindful of the type and amount of carbohydrates consumed, focusing on those with lower glycemic indexes.

Remember, individual responses to foods can vary, so it's essential to monitor blood sugar levels regularly and consult with a healthcare professional or a registered dietitian for personalized advice.

Chapter 5 Meal Planning Strategies

To help control blood sugar levels through meal planning:

Choose Complex Carbs: Opt for whole grains, legumes, and vegetables over refined carbohydrates to promote stable blood sugar.

Balanced Meals: Include a balance of carbohydrates, proteins, and healthy fats in each meal to slow down digestion and minimize blood sugar spikes.

Portion Control: Monitor portion sizes to avoid overeating, which can impact blood sugar levels. Use smaller plates if necessary.

Fiber-Rich Foods: Incorporate high-fiber foods like fruits, vegetables, and whole grains to help regulate blood sugar levels.

Lean Proteins: Include lean sources of protein, such as poultry, fish, tofu, and legumes, to help manage blood sugar.

Healthy Fats: Choose sources of healthy fats, like avocados, nuts, and olive oil, to support overall health and stabilize blood sugar.

Regular Meals: Aim for consistent meal times to establish a routine that can help regulate blood sugar levels.

Limit Processed Foods: Reduce the intake of processed foods, sugary snacks, and sugary beverages, as they can cause rapid blood sugar fluctuations.

Stay Hydrated: Drink plenty of water throughout the day to support overall health and aid digestion.

Monitor Blood Sugar Levels: Regularly check your blood sugar levels to understand how different foods affect you and make adjustments accordingly.

Smart snacking: involves making mindful choices to support overall health and maintain stable blood sugar levels. Opt for snacks that combine protein, healthy fats, and complex carbohydrates to provide sustained energy. Examples include nuts, Greek yogurt with berries, or whole grain crackers with hummus. To stabilize blood sugar, avoid sugary snacks and refined carbohydrates. Instead, focus on portion control and eat smaller, balanced snacks throughout the day. Include fiber-rich foods like fruits, vegetables, and whole grains to help regulate blood sugar levels. Stay hydrated, as dehydration can impact blood sugar.

Listen to your body's hunger and fullness cues, and plan snacks ahead to avoid reaching for unhealthy options when hunger strikes. Regular meals and snacks spaced evenly throughout the day can contribute to better blood sugar control.

Always consult with a healthcare professional or a registered dietitian for personalized advice based on your specific health needs and goals.

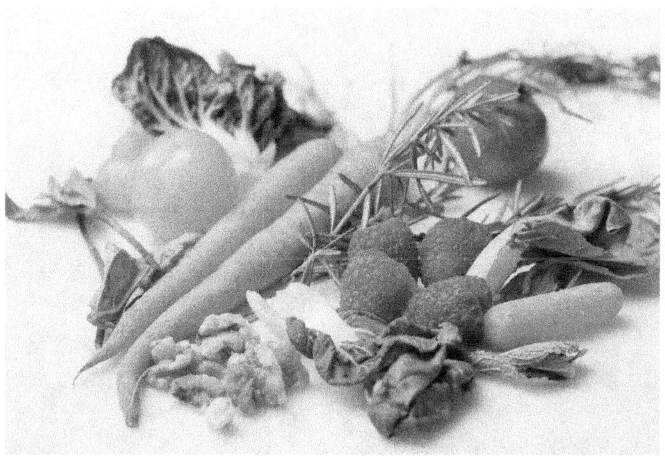

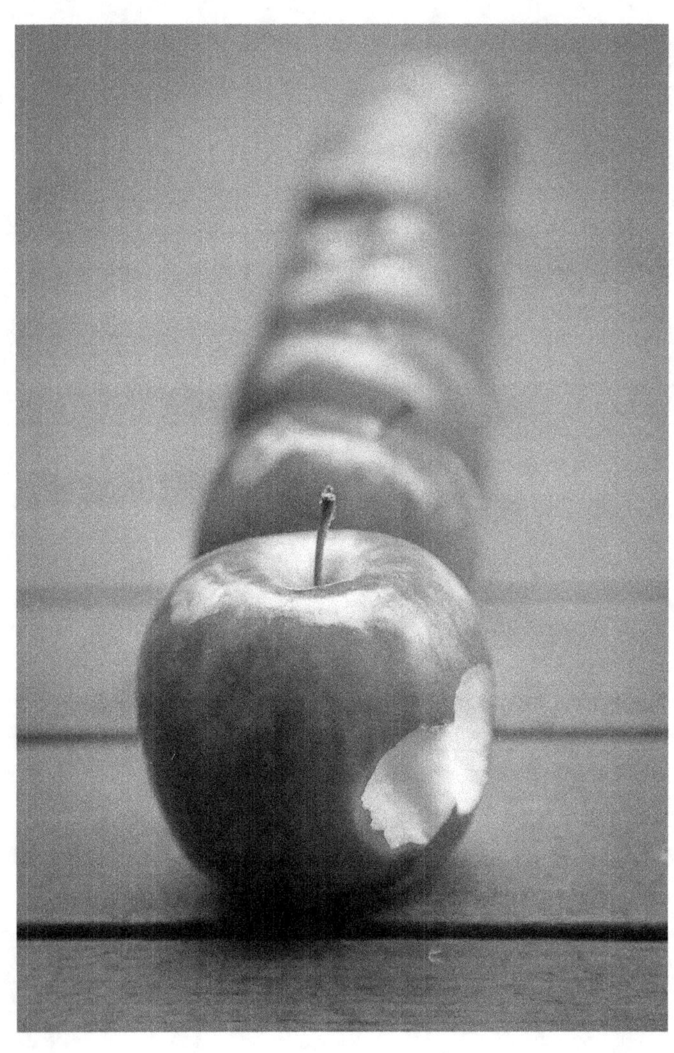

Chapter 6 – The power of hydration

Hydration plays a crucial role in blood sugar control as it helps regulate glucose levels in several ways. Firstly, adequate water intake supports the kidneys in flushing out excess glucose through urine, contributing to stable blood sugar levels. Additionally, proper hydration ensures efficient transport of nutrients, including glucose, in the bloodstream.

Moreover, dehydration can lead to concentrated blood, making glucose levels more difficult to manage. Staying well-hydrated promotes optimal circulation, aiding the body in utilizing insulin effectively. Consistent hydration also supports overall metabolic function, which is essential for maintaining balanced blood sugar.

Certain beverages can impact blood sugar levels. Sugary drinks, like sodas and fruit juices, can cause a rapid spike in blood sugar. Opting for water, herbal teas, or beverages without added sugars can be a better choice to help maintain stable blood sugar levels. It's essential for individuals with diabetes or those watching their

blood sugar to be mindful of their beverage
choices.

In summary, the power of hydration in blood sugar
control lies in its ability to assist kidney function,
optimize nutrient transport, and promote efficient
insulin activity, emphasizing the importance of
staying adequately hydrated for overall health.

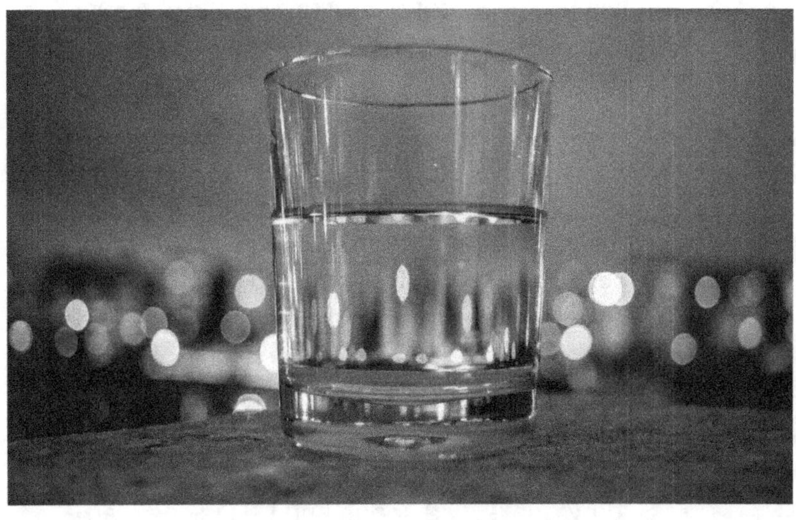

Chapter 7 – Lifestyle Factors - Blood sugar control lifestyle

Maintaining stable blood sugar levels is crucial for overall health. Lifestyle factors play a key role in blood sugar control. These include:

Diet: Choose complex carbohydrates with a low glycemic index as discussed in the previous chapters, Include fiber-rich foods to slow down sugar absorption.

Control portion sizes to manage calorie intake.

Physical Activity: Regular exercise helps insulin work more efficiently.

Both aerobic exercises and strength training contribute to blood sugar control.

Weight Management: Achieving and maintaining a healthy weight reduces insulin resistance.

Even a modest weight loss can have a significant impact.

Stress Management: Chronic stress can elevate blood sugar levels.

Practices such as meditation, deep breathing, or yoga can help manage stress.

Sleep Quality: Lack of sleep can affect insulin sensitivity. Aim for 7-9 hours of quality sleep each night.

Hydration: Proper hydration supports kidney function in regulating blood sugar.
Water is the best choice; limit sugary beverages.

Regular Monitoring: Regularly check blood sugar levels as advised by healthcare professionals. Monitoring helps in understanding how lifestyle choices impact blood sugar.

Alcohol Consumption: Consume alcohol in moderation, as it can affect blood sugar levels. Avoid excessive drinking, especially on an empty stomach.

Smoking Cessation: Smoking increases the risk of diabetes complications. Quitting smoking improves overall health and can positively impact blood sugar.
Medication Adherence: If prescribed medication, take it as directed by healthcare professionals. Consult with healthcare providers before making any changes.
By incorporating these lifestyle factors into daily routines, individuals can contribute to better blood sugar management and overall well-being.

Chapter 8 Blood sugar symphony

Monitoring and adjusting blood sugar levels is a delicate dance, akin to orchestrating a symphony of metabolic harmony within the body. Picture a vigilant conductor, the glucometer, wielding its baton to extract the precise notes of glucose concentration from a single drop of blood. The orchestral players, insulin and glucagon, respond to this maestro's cues, modulating their rhythms to maintain equilibrium.

Yet, this symphony is not without its unpredictable crescendos and diminuendos. A vigilant eye must be cast upon the musical score, the blood glucose readings, as they flutter in real-time. Like a skilled composer, the individual must interpret these notes and decide when to adjust the tempo – perhaps with a calculated bolus of insulin or a measured intake of carbohydrates.

In this intricate ballet, the body's responses are the choreography, and the individual becomes both dancer and choreographer. The grace lies in the ability to adapt, to intuitively sense when the blood sugar melody is veering off-key and to make swift adjustments to restore harmony.

Imagine a tightrope walker traversing the thin line between hyperglycemia and hypoglycemia. Each step is a decision, a moment of calibration, where the walker adjusts their balance – a metaphor for adjusting insulin doses, altering meal plans, or incorporating physical activity into the routine.

The visual narrative of blood sugar control extends beyond numbers on a screen; it is a living canvas painted with the hues of resilience, discipline, and adaptation. It's the art of balancing the body's metabolic brushstrokes to create a masterpiece of health and well-being.

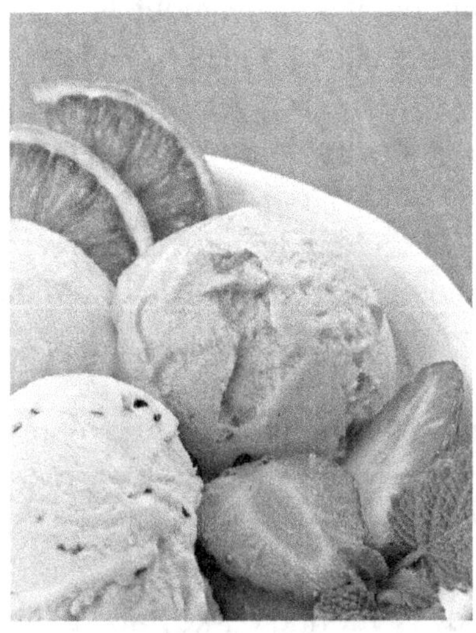

Chapter 9 – Recipes for Blood Sugar Control (Breakfast, lunch and dinner ideas) and Healthy dessert options for blood sugar

In this chapter we will be discussing briefly on Balanced Recipe for Blood Sugar Control with emphasis on breakfast, lunch and dinner ideas haven't discussed extensively on crafting and balancing diets in the previous chapters as Balancing your meals is crucial for blood sugar control.

For breakfast: try a bowl of steel-cut oats topped with fresh berries and a sprinkle of chia seeds. This provides complex carbs and fiber for sustained energy.

At lunch: opt for a colorful salad with leafy greens, grilled chicken, cherry tomatoes, and a vinaigrette made with olive oil. Include a small portion of quinoa or brown rice for added fiber and protein.

For dinner: go for baked salmon with roasted sweet potatoes and steamed broccoli. The omega-3 fatty acids in salmon contribute to heart health, while sweet potatoes offer a slower release of energy.

Snack wisely with a handful of mixed nuts or Greek yogurt with sliced almonds. These snacks provide healthy fats and protein, helping to keep blood sugar levels stable between meals.

Remember to monitor portion sizes, and consider spreading your meals throughout the day to prevent drastic spikes or drops in blood sugar. Always consult with a healthcare professional for personalized advice.

Healthy Dessert Options for blood Sugar

Opting for desserts that are low in added sugars and rich in fiber can be beneficial for blood sugar control. Consider incorporating the following healthy dessert options:

Fresh Fruit Salad: Packed with vitamins, minerals, and fiber.
Choose fruits with lower glycemic index, such as berries, cherries, and apples.

Greek Yogurt Parfait: Greek yogurt is high in protein and lower in carbohydrates.
Layer it with fresh fruits, nuts, and a drizzle of honey for natural sweetness.

Chia Seed Pudding: Chia seeds are rich in fiber and omega-3 fatty acids.
Mix with unsweetened almond milk and let it sit to form a pudding. Top with berries.

Baked Apples with Cinnamon: Apples contain fiber and natural sweetness.
Sprinkle with cinnamon, which may help regulate blood sugar.

Avocado Chocolate Mousse: Avocado adds a creamy texture with healthy fats.
Mix with cocoa powder and a sweetener like stevia or monk fruit.

Sugar-Free Sorbet: Make sorbet using natural fruit flavors without added sugars.
Blend frozen fruits like berries or mango with a splash of water.

Nuts and Seeds Energy Bites: Combine nuts, seeds, and a natural sweetener like dates or honey.

Form into bite-sized portions for a satisfying treat.

Coconut Yogurt with Berries: Coconut yogurt is a dairy-free option with a creamy texture.
Top with fresh berries for added antioxidants.

Dark Chocolate-Covered Almonds: Dark chocolate in moderation contains less sugar.
Pair it with almonds for a satisfying mix of sweetness and crunch.

Baked Oatmeal Cups: Use rolled oats, mashed banana, and a small amount of natural sweetener.
Customize with nuts, seeds, or berries.
Remember to monitor portion sizes, as even healthy desserts can impact blood sugar levels if consumed excessively. It's also advisable to consult with a healthcare professional or a nutritionist for personalized advice based on individual health needs.

Chapter 10
Diabetic-Friendly Eating Guide and Addressing Challenges and Cravings

Diabetic-friendly eating is essential for managing blood sugar levels and promoting overall health in individuals with diabetes. The key principles revolve around balanced nutrition, mindful food choices, and portion control. Here are some comprehensive guidelines:

1. **Carbohydrate Management**:
Choose Complex Carbs: Opt for whole grains, legumes, vegetables, and fruits with a low glycemic index to prevent rapid spikes in blood sugar.
Portion Control: Monitor carbohydrate intake and distribute it evenly throughout the day to maintain stable blood sugar levels.

2. **Protein-Rich Foods:**
Lean Proteins: Incorporate lean sources like poultry, fish, tofu, legumes, and low-fat dairy to help manage blood sugar without causing spikes.

3. Healthy Fats:

Good Fats: Include sources of healthy fats, such as avocados, nuts, seeds, and olive oil, to support heart health and provide sustained energy.

4. **Fiber Intake**:

High-Fiber Foods: Consume fiber-rich foods like vegetables, fruits, whole grains, and legumes to aid digestion and help control blood sugar levels.

5. **Portion Control**:

Balanced Meals: Opt for balanced meals that include a combination of carbohydrates, proteins, and fats. Pay attention to portion sizes to avoid overeating.

6. **Regular Meal Timing**:

Consistent Schedule: Stick to a regular eating schedule with evenly spaced meals to regulate blood sugar levels and avoid extreme highs or lows.

7. **Limit Added Sugars**:

Read Labels: Be vigilant about food labels to identify hidden sugars in processed foods and beverages. Opt for natural sweeteners or limit sugar intake.

8. **Hydration**:

Water is Key: Stay well-hydrated with water as the primary beverage. Limit sugary drinks and alcohol, as they can impact blood sugar levels.

9. **Monitoring Blood Sugar**:

Regular Testing: Monitor blood sugar levels as advised by healthcare professionals. Regular testing helps in understanding how different foods affect your body.

10. **Individualized Approach**: Work with a healthcare team, including a dietitian, to create an individualized meal plan based on your specific needs, preferences, and lifestyle.

11. **Physical Activity**: Regular Exercise: Incorporate regular physical activity into your routine, as it can improve insulin sensitivity and help control blood sugar levels.

12. **Healthy Cooking Methods**: Grilling, Baking, Steaming: Opt for healthier cooking methods to retain nutritional value without adding excess fats.

13. **Mindful Eating:** Slow, Enjoyable Meals: Practice mindful eating by savoring each bite, chewing slowly, and paying attention to hunger and fullness cues.

14. **Educational Resources**: Stay Informed: Continuously educate yourself about diabetes management, nutrition, and lifestyle changes. Stay updated on the latest research and recommendations.

Remember, individual responses to foods may vary, so it's crucial to consult with healthcare professionals for personalized guidance. Regular monitoring and adjustments to your diet based on your body's responses are key elements in effective diabetes management.

Addressing Challenges and cravings in blood sugar control

Managing blood sugar levels poses several challenges, particularly for individuals with diabetes or those at risk of developing the condition. One primary challenge is the need for consistent monitoring. Regular blood glucose testing is crucial to understanding one's levels and making informed decisions about diet, medication, and lifestyle. The craving for high-sugar foods can complicate this process, as individuals may struggle to resist temptations that can lead to spikes in blood sugar.

Dietary choices play a pivotal role in blood sugar control. The challenge lies in striking a balance between enjoying a satisfying and nutritious diet while avoiding excessive carbohydrates and sugars. Cravings for sugary snacks or comfort foods can be intense, making it difficult for individuals to adhere to a diabetes-friendly diet. Overcoming these cravings often requires a combination of willpower, education on healthier food alternatives, and support from healthcare professionals or support groups.

Another challenge is the impact of stress on blood sugar levels. Stress triggers the release of hormones that can cause a rise in blood glucose.

Managing stress is essential, but in today's fast-paced world, this is often easier said than done. Techniques such as mindfulness, regular exercise, and adequate sleep can contribute to stress reduction, positively influencing blood sugar control.

Consistency in medication and insulin management is critical, but factors like forgetfulness or fear of injections can pose challenges. Educating individuals on the importance of adhering to prescribed medications and addressing concerns can help overcome these obstacles. Additionally, financial constraints or lack of access to healthcare may hinder the consistent acquisition of necessary medications or monitoring supplies.

Physical activity is a cornerstone of diabetes management, yet incorporating regular exercise into a busy lifestyle can be challenging. Finding enjoyable forms of exercise and integrating them into daily routines can be a solution, but time constraints and physical limitations may still pose obstacles.

Social situations and peer pressure can also be challenging. Attending events with tempting food options or facing societal norms that encourage unhealthy eating can make it difficult to stick to a diabetes-friendly lifestyle. Building a strong support system of friends, family, or community groups can provide encouragement and understanding in these situations and as such, achieving and maintaining optimal blood sugar control involves navigating a complex interplay of dietary choices, stress management, medication adherence, physical activity, and social influences. Recognizing and addressing these challenges, along with cultivating a proactive and informed approach to diabetes management, can significantly improve outcomes and overall well-being

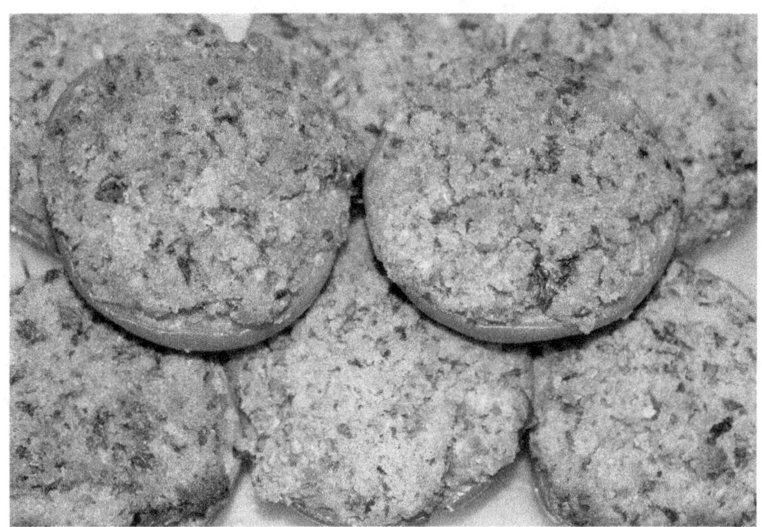

• Conclusion

In conclusion, the dietary solution presented in this book offers a comprehensive and evidence-based approach to managing blood sugar levels. By emphasizing a balanced and nutrient-dense diet, readers are empowered to make informed choices that can positively impact their overall health and well-being.

The integration of whole foods, particularly those with a low glycemic index, plays a pivotal role in stabilizing blood sugar levels. The emphasis on lean proteins, fiber-rich vegetables, and healthy fats not only supports glucose regulation but also fosters sustained energy throughout the day.

Furthermore, the incorporation of mindful eating practices and portion control enhances the effectiveness of this dietary solution. By promoting awareness of hunger and satiety cues, individuals can establish a healthier relationship with food, mitigating the risk of overconsumption and subsequent blood sugar spikes.

The inclusion of practical tips and meal plans tailored to different dietary preferences ensures that the approach presented in this book is accessible and adaptable to a diverse range of lifestyles. This flexibility encourages long-term adherence, fostering sustainable habits that contribute to improved blood sugar management.

It is essential to recognize that dietary interventions are most effective when combined with regular physical activity and a holistic approach to health. Readers are encouraged to consult with healthcare professionals to tailor the dietary recommendations to their specific needs and medical conditions.

Ultimately, this dietary solution serves as a valuable resource for individuals seeking a proactive and empowering strategy to regulate blood sugar levels. By embracing the principles outlined in this book, readers have the opportunity to take control of their health and embark on a journey toward sustained well-being.

DIETARY TIME TABLE

Days	Breakfast	Lunch	Dinner
1			
2			
3			
4			

5			
6			
7			
8			
9			
10			

11

12

13

14

15

16

17			46
18			
19			

•